The Science of Senses

How Animals SMELL

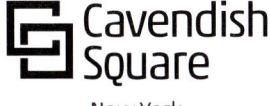
New York

Alicia Z. Klepeis

Published in 2019 by Cavendish Square Publishing, LLC
243 5th Avenue, Suite 136, New York, NY 10016

Copyright © 2019 by Cavendish Square Publishing, LLC

First Edition

No part of this publication may be reproduced, stored in a retrieval system, or transmitted in any form or by any means—electronic, mechanical, photocopying, recording, or otherwise—without the prior permission of the copyright owner. Request for permission should be addressed to Permissions, Cavendish Square Publishing, 243 5th Avenue, Suite 136, New York, NY 10016. Tel (877) 980-4450; fax (877) 980-4454.

Website: cavendishsq.com

This publication represents the opinions and views of the author based on his or her personal experience, knowledge, and research. The information in this book serves as a general guide only. The author and publisher have used their best efforts in preparing this book and disclaim liability rising directly or indirectly from the use and application of this book.

All websites were available and accurate when this book was sent to press.

Library of Congress Cataloging-in-Publication Data

Names: Klepeis, Alicia, 1971- author.
Title: How animals smell / Alicia Z. Klepeis.
Description: First edition. | New York : Cavendish Square, 2019. | Series: The science of senses |
Audience: Grades 2-5. | Includes bibliographical references and index.
Identifiers: LCCN 2018024024 (print) | LCCN 2018025456 (ebook) | ISBN 9781502642110 (ebook) |
ISBN 9781502642103 (library bound) | ISBN 9781502642080 (paperback) | ISBN 9781502642097 (6 pack)
Subjects: LCSH: Smell--Juvenile literature. | Senses and sensation--Juvenile literature. | Animals--Juvenile literature.
Classification: LCC QP458 (ebook) | LCC QP458 .K547 2019 (print) | DDC 612.8/6--dc23
LC record available at https://lccn.loc.gov/2018024024

Editorial Director: David McNamara
Editor: Kristen Susienka
Copy Editor: Nathan Heidelberger
Associate Art Director: Alan Sliwinski
Designer: Ginny Kemmerer
Production Coordinator: Karol Szymczuk
Photo Research: J8 Media

The photographs in this book are used by permission and through the courtesy of: Cover Ashwin/illusive.in/Moment Open/Getty Images; p. 4 Logoboom/Shutterstock.com; p. 6 Zairiazmal/Shutterstock.com; p. 7 (Top) Erwin Sparreboom/Shutterstock.com, (Bottom) Agnieszka Bacal/Shutterstock.com; p. 8 Reptiles4all/Shutterstock.com; p. 10 (Top) Barrett Hedges/National Geographic/Getty Images, (Bottom) Ondrej Prosicky/Shutterstock.com; p. 11 Sven Gruse/EyeEm/Getty Images (Top) Charlesjsharp/Sharp Photography (http://www.sharpphotography.co.uk/)/File: Meerkat (Suricata suricatta) Tswalu.jpg/Wikimedia Commons/CCA-SA 4.0 International (Center) Florence Gabriel/EyeEm/Getty Images; (Bottom) p. 12 Ekaterina Kolomeets/Shutterstock.com; p. 14 Jacopin/BSIP SA/Alamy Stock Photo; p. 15 SJ Allen/Shutterstock.com; p. 17 Alexander Safonov/Moment/Getty Images; p. 18 Michael Sheehan/EyeEm/Getty Images; p. 19 Oakley Originals/File: Dog nose 0002.jpg/Wikimedia Commons/CCA-2.0 Generic; p. 20 3bugsmom/Istockphoto.com; p. 23 Judy Kennamer/Shutterstock.com; p. 24 Paul Bradbury/OJO Images/Getty Images; p. 27 Xavier Rossi/Gamma-Rapho/Getty Images.

Printed in the United States of America

CONTENTS

One An Introduction to Smell 5

Two The Science of Smelling 13

Three People Versus Animals 21

Glossary 28

Find Out More 29

Index 31

About the Author 32

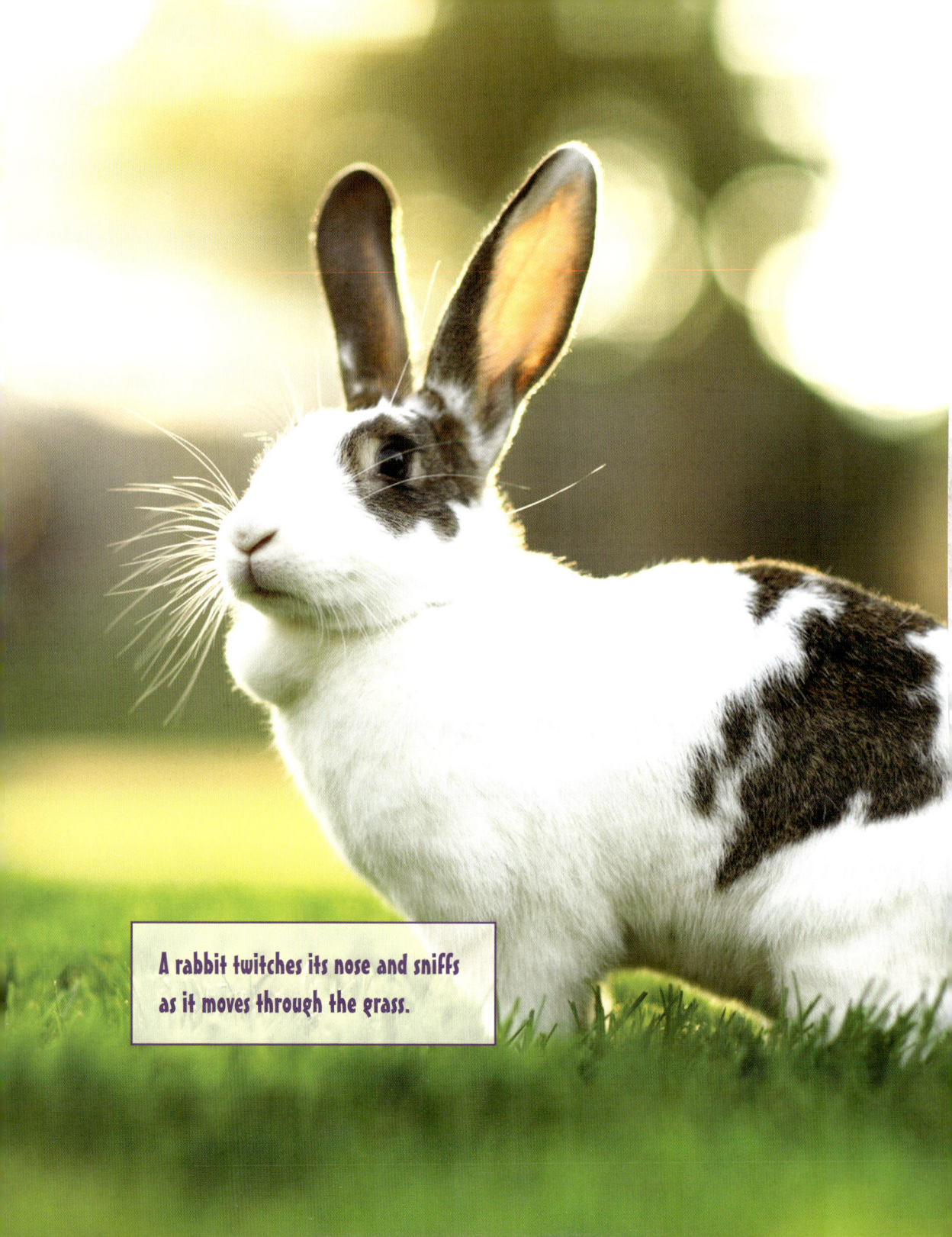

A rabbit twitches its nose and sniffs as it moves through the grass.

Chapter One

An Introduction to Smell

The sense of smell is very important for animals. It helps animals find food. It helps animals find a mate or find their babies. Smell also helps animals avoid being eaten by predators. The sense of smell tells animals about the world around them.

Why Smell Is Important

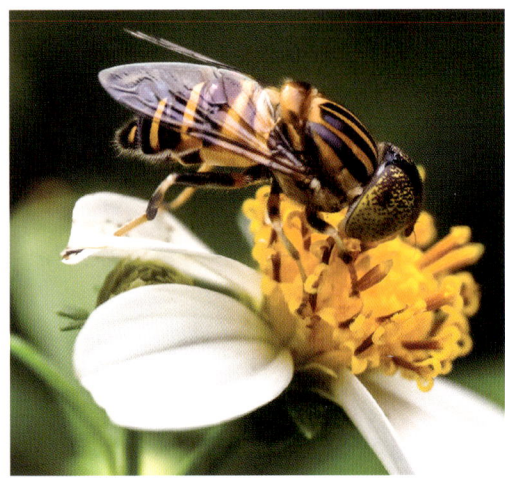

A hover fly sucks nectar from a flower. Hover flies often visit gardens to find food.

Where an animal lives and what it eats helps an animal's sense of smell develop.

Let's look at hover flies. Hover flies look like bees. They don't sting. They like to drink from flowers. They use smell to choose a flower to drink from.

Different Ways of Smelling

Many animals use their noses to smell. However, some animals don't. They use other body parts to smell.

Birds have **nostrils** just like people. Most birds have nostrils on their beaks. The bird uses its nostrils to sniff

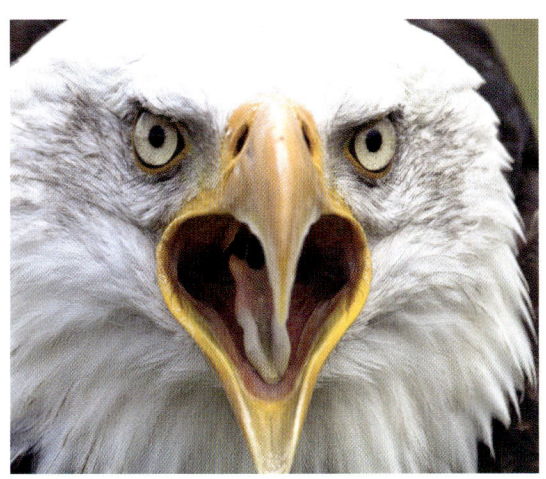

This close-up of a bald eagle shows its nostrils, located at the base of its large beak.

and smell. The sense of smell helps birds fly. It acts like a road map for birds. It helps them travel the skies.

The star-nosed mole has one of the weirdest noses on Earth. It has twenty-two **rays** around its nostrils. These rays move as the mole moves underground, where it lives. They help it look for food. The star-nosed mole can even smell underwater. It blows out air bubbles and sucks them back into its nose.

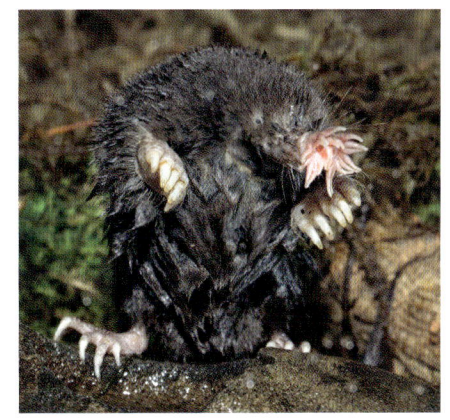

This image shows the pink rays around the star-nosed mole's nostrils. It also shows the mole's very sharp claws.

An Introduction to Smell

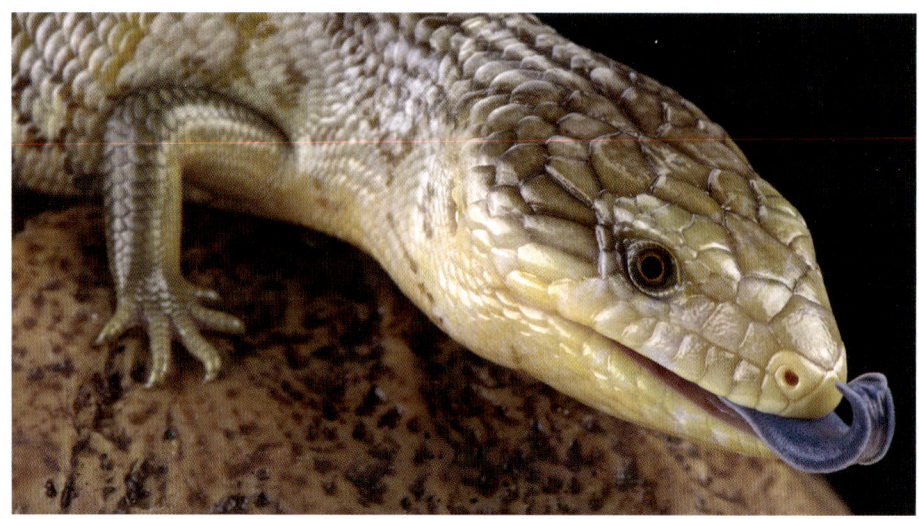

A Tanimbar blue-tongued skink uses its colorful tongue to smell. This reptile is found in Indonesia.

Snakes and lizards use their tongues to smell. They flick their tongues in and out. This lets them smell around them. Smells might tell a hungry snake where to find food. They might also help a lizard avoid an enemy.

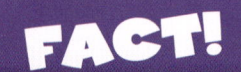

Some animals cannot smell. Examples include whales, dolphins, and porpoises.

FACT!

Male moths can smell female moths over 1 mile (1.6 kilometers) away. They use their antennae to smell them.

Butterflies have an excellent sense of smell. They smell with their **antennae** and legs. They have organs there. The organs help them smell. Butterflies can smell when nectar is flowing from flowers.

An octopus uses the suckers that run up and down its arms to smell. These suckers are like hands that can smell and taste. An octopus might stick an arm into a crack to see what is hiding inside.

ANIMALS AROUND THE WORLD

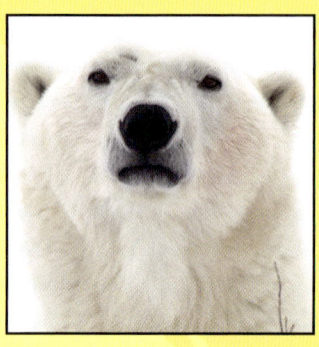

NORTH AMERICA: A polar bear's nose is so powerful it can smell a seal under 3 feet (0.9 meters) of ice!

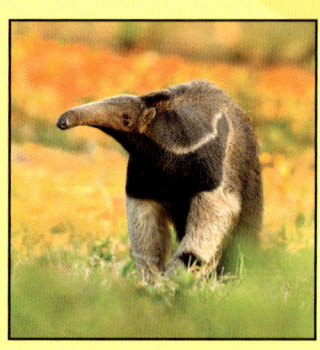

CENTRAL AND SOUTH AMERICA: The sense of smell of the giant anteater is forty times better than a human's sense of smell.

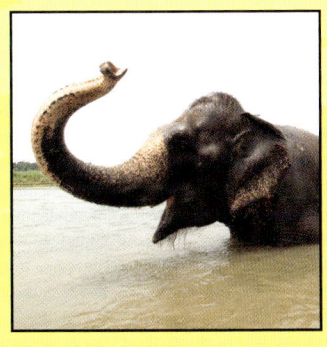

ASIA: Asian elephants are amazing at smelling water. They can smell it underground and far away. They can smell it from 12 miles (19 km) away.

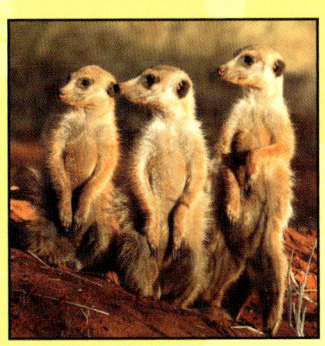

AFRICA: Meerkats can smell food (like rodents or insects) underground.

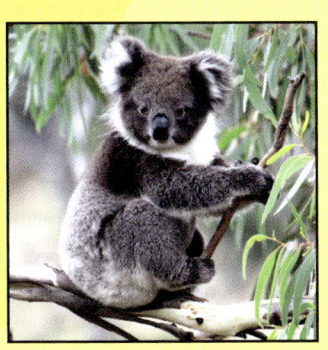

AUSTRALIA: A koala's powerful sense of smell helps it tell the difference between different kinds of eucalyptus plants.

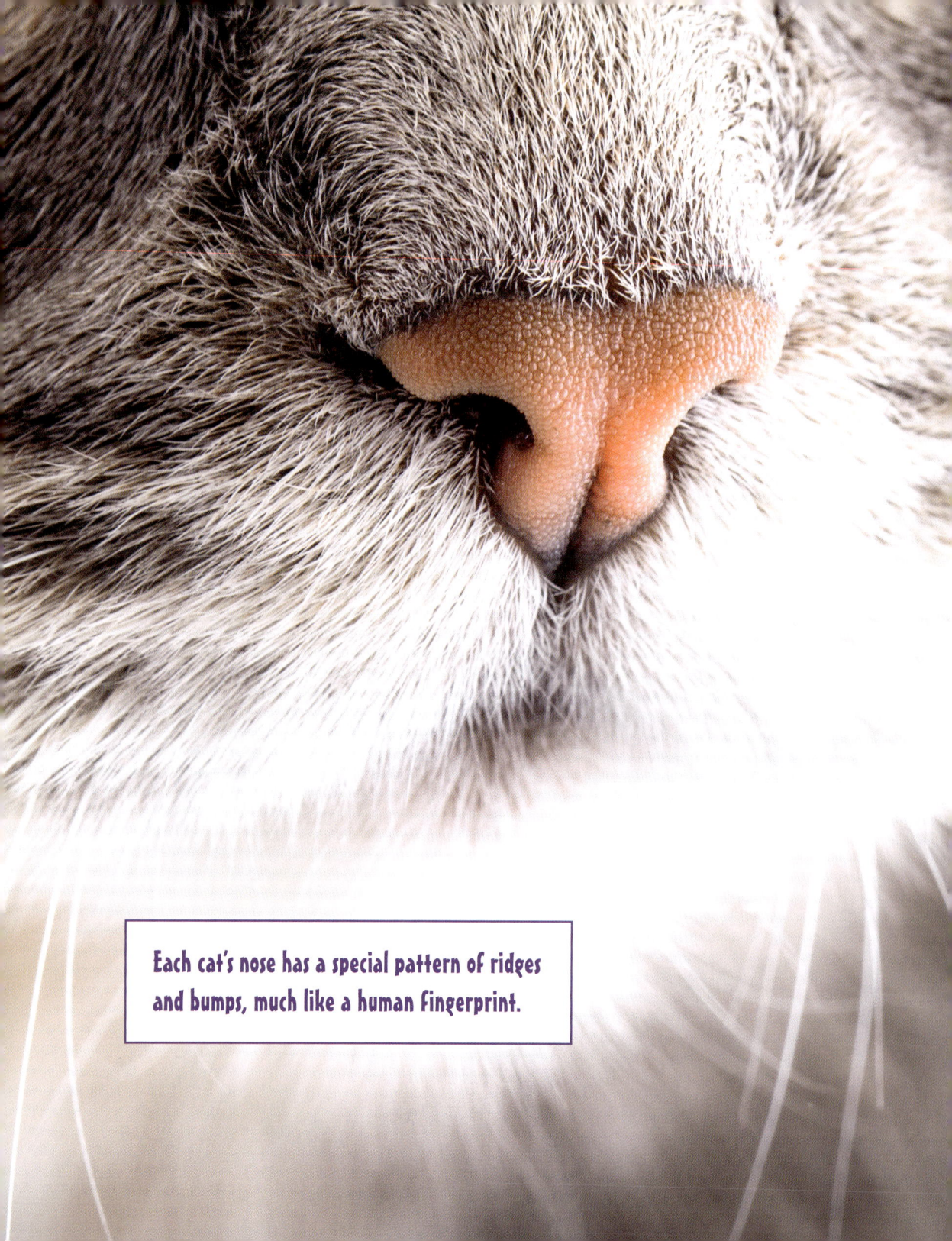

Each cat's nose has a special pattern of ridges and bumps, much like a human fingerprint.

Chapter Two

The Science of Smelling

Animals use their sense of smell every day. But how does the sense of smell work?

How Do Animals Smell?

Most animals smell with their noses. A cat is one example. A cat's nose is close to the ground. The cat can pick up all kinds of smells with its nose. It can smell fast food from wrappers left behind, a blooming flower, and another cat that rubbed up against a tree nearby.

Most objects around us have a scent. The wrappers or flowers the cat smelled had a scent on them. Scents are made up of tiny **molecules**. Usually molecules are light. They can float through the air. To smell something, molecules have to reach an animal's nose. Inside the nose are an animal's **scent receptors**.

A scent receptor passes information to other cells that help the animal smell. These cells are called an **olfactory bulb**. This is part of the brain. It receives information

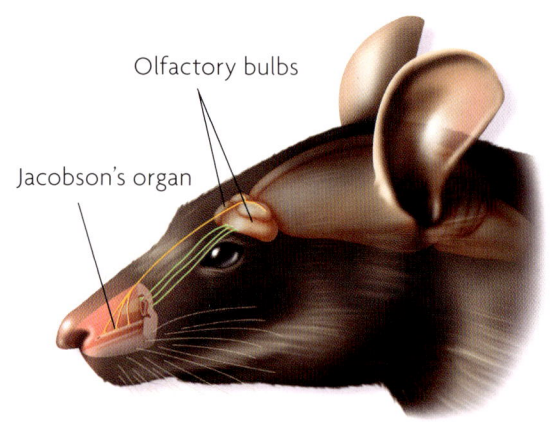

Olfactory bulbs

Jacobson's organ

This diagram shows a rat's Jacobson's organ and how that organ is connected to the brain. The Jacobson's organ is part of the animal's smelling system.

about scents from the nose. Then it passes the information on to other parts of the animal's brain. The brain tells the animal what the smell is.

A Special Smell

Cats and other animals have a special part of their bodies. The body part is called the Jacobson's organ. It is on the roof of the animal's mouth. It helps the animal smell better. When a cat or other animal smells something new or different, it might open its mouth. That means the animal is smelling the

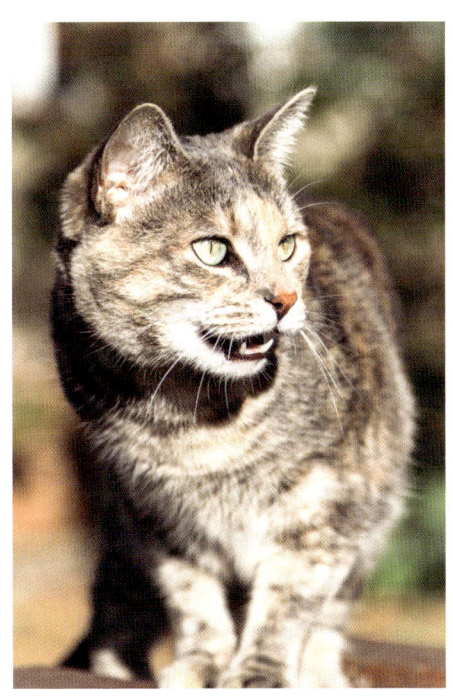

The mouth of this tabby cat is open, allowing the cat to use its Jacobson's organ to smell.

> **FACT!**
> Some animals use smell to mark their territory or warn off enemies. Examples include skunk spray and cheetah urine.

object with the Jacobson's organ. It uses this organ whenever it thinks a smell needs extra investigating. Examples of other animals with a Jacobson's organ include rats, pigs, tigers, and snakes.

Shark Sniffers

Underwater animals smell things too. A shark is one example. A shark glides along the ocean. Water flows through the shark's nostrils. These are located on the underside of its snout. The water comes into the shark's nostrils. Like air, water can carry scent molecules. Inside the nostrils are cells that pick up the scent.

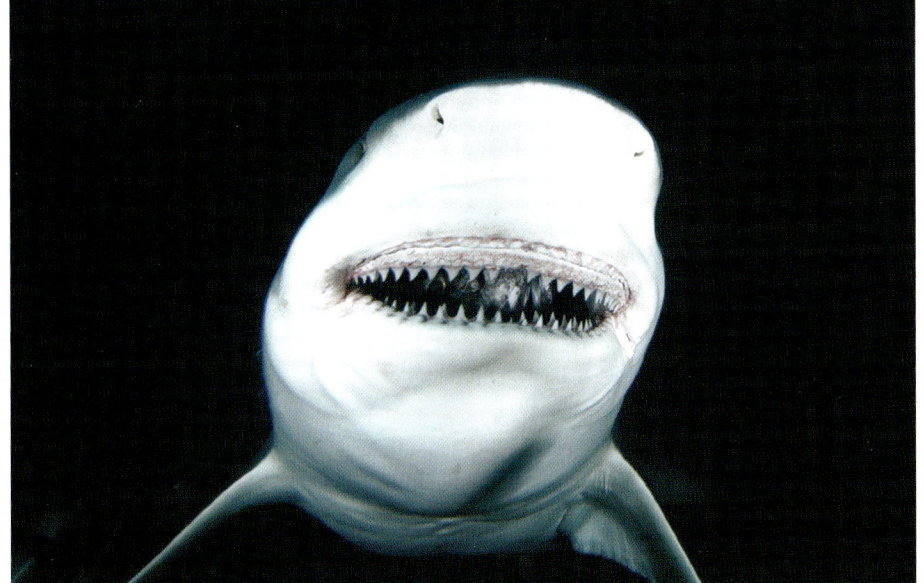

A bull shark takes in many scents as it swims through the Beqa Lagoon of Fiji. Its nostrils are located on the underside of its snout.

Signals are sent to the shark's brain. The shark's brain interprets these signals as smells.

A shark's nose just has one purpose: to smell. Sharks don't breathe through their noses. They breathe through their gills. As much as 40 percent of a shark's

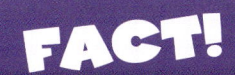

A great white shark could smell one drop of blood in an Olympic-sized pool!

brain is dedicated to its sense of smell. Because of their great sense of smell, sharks are sometimes called "swimming noses."

Best Sniffers in the Animal Kingdom

Some animals have extremely good senses of smell. Which creatures are super sniffers? Elephants top the list. They have 2,000 **genes** dedicated to smell. Other animals have great senses of smell too. Rats take second place. They have about 1,200 genes dedicated to scent. Cows, mice, and horses are also good sniffers. Dogs come in sixth. And humans? People have less than 400 genes devoted to scent.

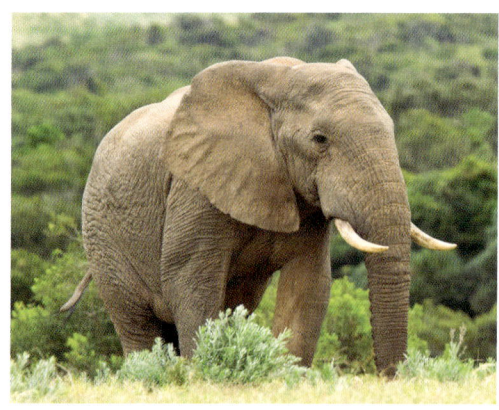

An elephant stands in a grassy field. Elephants use smell both to identify family members and to find food.

A DOG'S SENSE OF SMELL

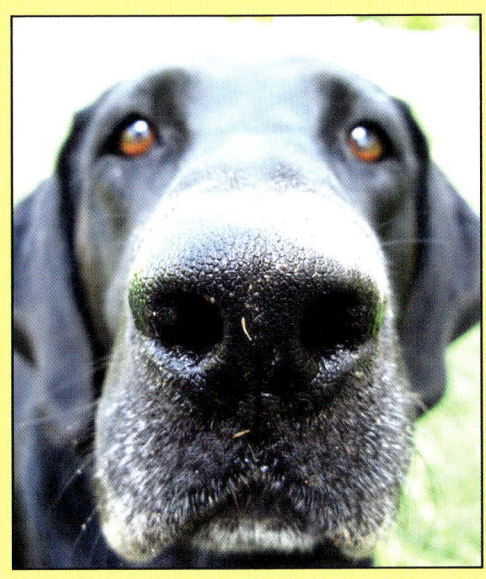

This close-up shows the shape of a dog's nostrils. Their shape is part of why dogs are such good smellers.

Dogs have an amazing sense of smell. Their nostrils are shaped like commas. This shape helps the air swirl in as it enters the dog's nose. Scent molecules can better move around once inside the nose. Dogs can also flare their nostrils to bring in more air.

Dogs can move each of their nostrils separately. This helps them figure out which direction a smell is coming from.

The Science of Smelling

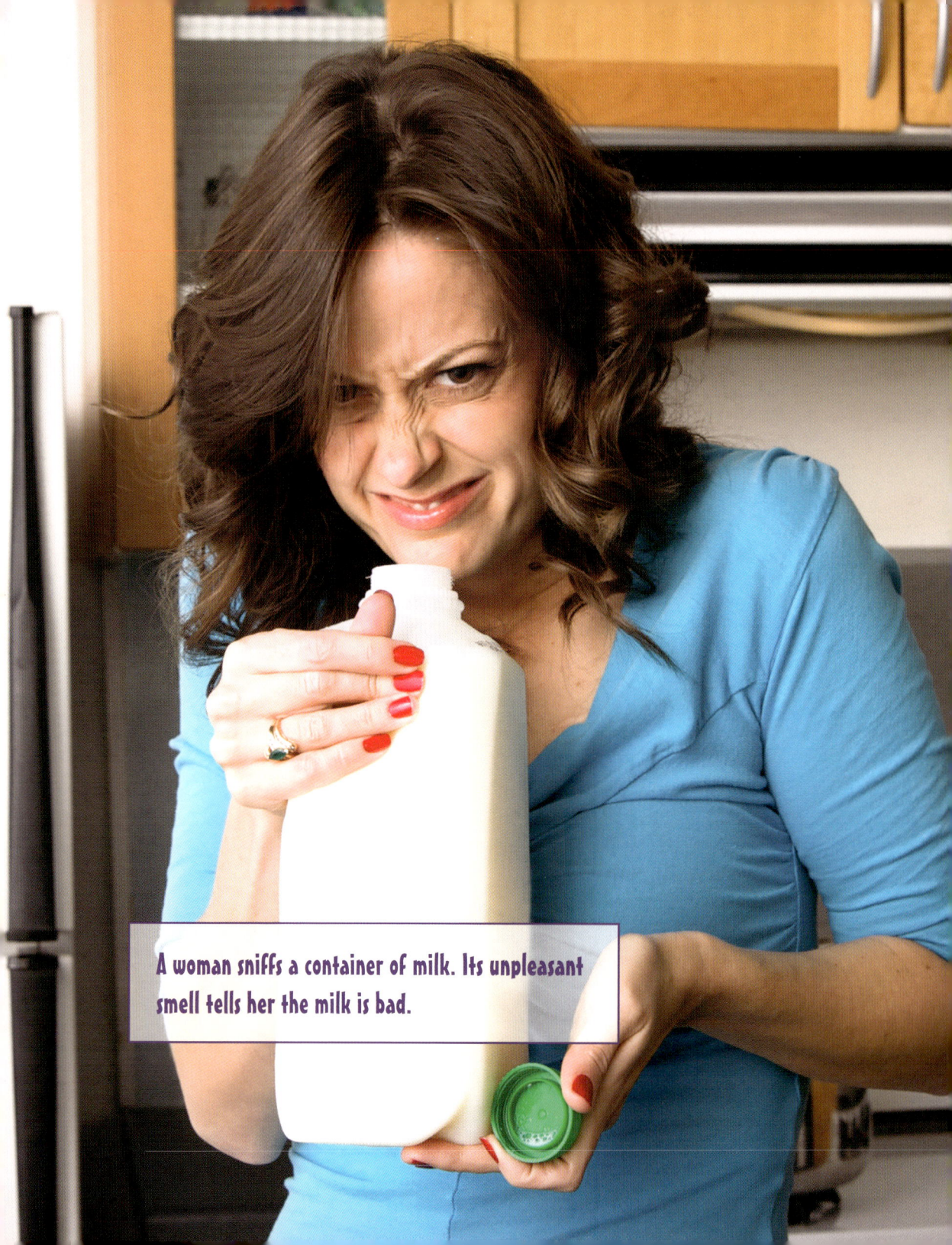

A woman sniffs a container of milk. Its unpleasant smell tells her the milk is bad.

Chapter Three

People Versus Animals

Just like other animals, people have a sense of smell. You use this sense every day. Maybe you sniff a week-old container of milk to see if it's still OK to drink. Your nose may also tell you that your baby brother is ready for a diaper change.

> **FACT!**
> Research shows that women have a better sense of smell than men.

Humans' Sense of Smell Over Time

People's sense of smell developed over millions of years. Our early human ancestors used this sense for many things. It helped them stay away from rotten meat and poisonous plants. It let them sniff out good food sources. Smell even functioned as a tool to detect disease.

Smells have many impacts on people's lives. They can warn us of danger. Scents can help us remember old places or events. Scent can even help us remember people.

How Humans Smell

A man walks into a bakery. He smells sugary treats. What is happening inside him? First, the scent arrives at his nostrils. This scent is in the form of molecules. The scent travels into the man's **nasal passages**. These are located inside the body, behind the nose.

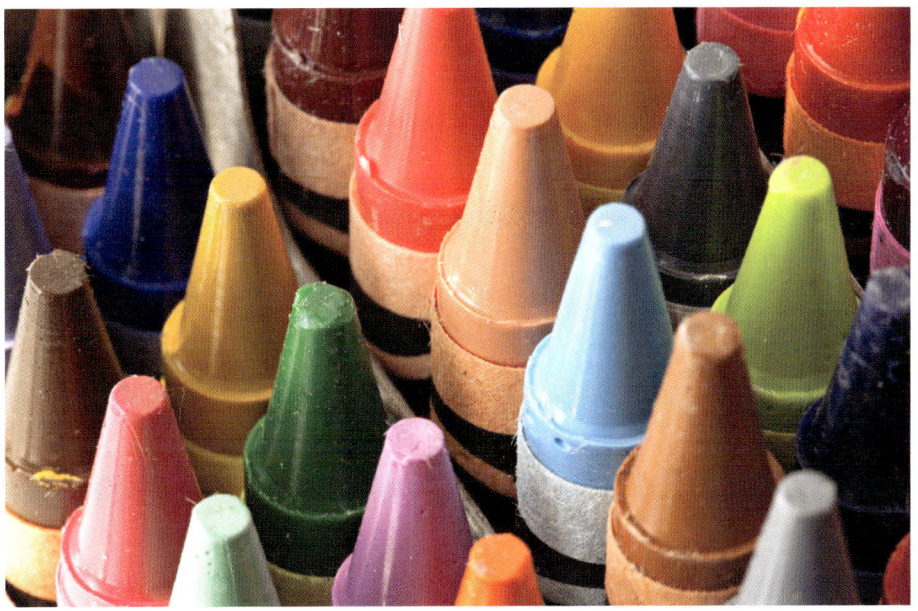

The smell of crayons has been proven to trigger memories and emotions in many people.

People Versus Animals 23

At the top of the nasal passages are scent receptors. They are made of cells called neurons. The air touches the neurons. Inside the nasal passages are hairlike structures. They are called cilia. Many animals have them too.

Scent molecules attach to the cilia. When this happens, the neurons pass information about the smell to the olfactory bulb. The olfactory bulb tells the person what the smell is. Yummy bread, in this case.

A young girl smells a flower in Cape Town, South Africa. Most people consider the scent of flowers to be pleasant.

Human Versus Animal Senses of Smell

Some of the ways people use their sense of smell

are the same as animals. Most people don't need to sniff underground to find hidden food. But they often smell food at the market or grocery store. Why? To figure out if a melon is ripe or rotten, for example. Many animals depend on their noses to determine what food is available and able to be eaten.

Animals may like or dislike the smell of other animals. This could be because the animal being sniffed is an enemy. Newborn animals can identify the scent of their mothers. This is true for rats and humans, for example.

Different but Still Great

In the past, many people believed that humans' sense of smell was worse than that of other animals. But new research is finding that to be false. A dog has more scent receptors than a person. But you can smell a banana just as well as a dog can. Humans can also track a scent

> **FACT!**
>
> **About two million people in the United States cannot smell. This condition is called anosmia.**

much like a dog. Scientists believe humans can sense as many as one trillion different scents.

Different animals' noses are tuned to focus on different things. People might be more sensitive than dogs to certain smells. Dogs might be more sensitive than people to other smells.

No matter what, the sense of smell tells animals all about the world in which they live. It seems that for animals and people, the nose knows!

SPECIAL RATS

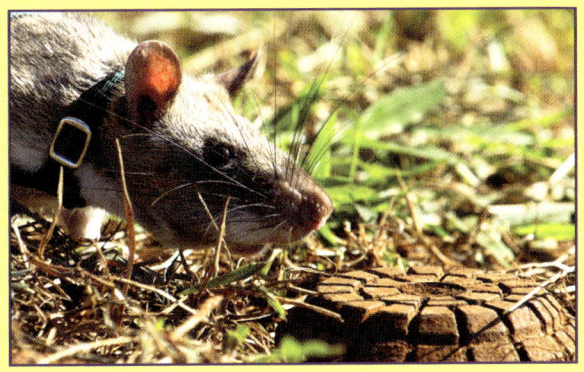

A trained sniffer rat tries to pinpoint the location of a land mine in the African country of Mozambique.

African giant pouched rats are cat-sized rodents. They have an awesome sense of smell. Today, these rats are working to discover hidden land mines. How? They can sniff out an explosive called TNT. One African giant pouched rat can search an area over 2,000 square feet (186 square meters) in only twenty minutes. That would take a human as long as four days.

GLOSSARY

antennae A thin pair of organs located on the heads of many bugs. They help bugs smell and feel around them.

genes Information a person (or animal) is born with that determines the person's looks and abilities.

molecules The smallest particles of a substance which have all the characteristics of that substance.

nasal passages Paths in the nose that help air flow through it.

nostrils Two openings in the nose that let animals breathe.

olfactory bulb A part of the brain that helps interpret smells.

rays Long tentacles used as sense organs.

scent receptors Specialized nerve cells that receive scents.

Find Out More

Books

Hewitt, Sally. *Smell*. Science in Action: My Senses. London: QEB Publishing, 2018.

Mangor, Jodie. *Animal Senses*. Vero Beach, FL: Rourke Publishing Group, 2017.

Rundgren, Helen. *The World's Best Noses, Ears, and Eyes*. New York: Holiday House, 2013.

Website

Amazing Animal Senses

https://faculty.washington.edu/chudler/amaze.html

This website provides information about some of the most amazing sensory abilities of all kinds of animals—from smell to taste to touch.

FIND OUT MORE CONTINUED

Videos

How Do Dogs "See" with Their Noses?

https://www.youtube.com/watch?v=p7fXa2Occ_U

This animated video clip shows how a dog's sense of smell works. It includes how a dog's sense of smell is different from a human's sense of smell.

How Your Nose Works Animation

https://www.youtube.com/watch?v=TJfGK87CMmk

This video shows how a person's sense of smell works from the time they breathe in air until their brain processes smells.

INDEX

Page numbers in **boldface** are illustrations. Entries in **boldface** are glossary terms.

antennae, 9
birds, 6–7, **7**
brain, 14–15, **14**, 17–18
cats, **12**, 13–15, **15**
cilia, 24
dogs, 18–19, **19**, 25–26
elephants, 11, **11**, 18, **18**
genes, 18
hover flies, 6, **6**
humans, 18, **20**, 21–26

Jacobson's organ, **14**, 15–16
molecules, 14, 16, 19, 23–24
nasal passages, 23–24
nostrils, 6–7, **7**, **12**, 16–17, **17**, 19, **19**, 23
octopuses, 9
olfactory bulb, 14–15, **14**, 24
rats, **14**, 16, 18, 25, 27, **27**
rays, 7, **7**
scent receptors, 14, 24–25
sharks, 16–18, **17**
star-nosed moles, 7, **7**
tongues, 8, **8**

Index   31

ABOUT THE AUTHOR

Alicia Z. Klepeis began her career at the National Geographic Society. Klepeis is the author of numerous children's and young adult books, including *Trolls*, *Engineering North America's Landmarks: Building Mount Rushmore*, and *A Time for Change*. Her favorite smells include hyacinth flowers and gummy bears.